# Trimming Pounds with Timed Fasting

Unlocking Weight Loss Through Intermittent Energy Restriction

# Evelyn C. Kohl

# Copyright

# About the author

Many people know Evelyn C. Kohl as a nutritionist and health writer who did groundbreaking work in the areas of diet and weight control. Evelyn has spent more than ten years studying how different diets affect people's health. She has a Master's degree in Nutrition Sciences from the University of California, Berkeley.

Her interest in eating began when she had trouble controlling her weight. This made her want to learn more about the science behind effective and long-lasting weight loss. Because of this, she became interested in intermittent energy restriction diets and has since done a lot of study on the topic.

When Evelyn dies, she focuses on finding a balance between science and reality. She thinks that changes to food should be based on science and be easy to incorporate into daily life. Her beliefs are based on the idea that losing weight shouldn't be a constant battle, but something that comes naturally and is fun.

"Trimming Pounds with Timed Fasting: Unlocking Weight Loss Through Intermittent Energy Restriction" is her most recent book. It is the result of many years of study and writing. Evelyn breaks down complicated nutritional ideas into simple words in this book so that a lot of people can understand it.

Apart from her writing, Evelyn is a sought-after speaker at health and wellness seminars, where she shares her views on nutrition and dieting. She also has a popular blog where she writes about health, diet, and everyday life.

Evelyn's work has been featured in several major health magazines and she has been a guest expert on various health-related TV and radio shows. Her commitment to supporting healthy and sustainable ways of living has made her a respected voice in the nutrition community.

# Table of content

# Introduction

## The Journey to a Lighter You

Welcome to "Trimming Pounds with Timed Fasting: Unlocking Weight Loss Through Intermittent Energy Restriction," a guide designed to revolutionize your understanding of dieting and help you start on a sustainable weight loss journey. In this book, we will explore the profound yet often misunderstood idea of intermittent energy restriction and how it can be a pivotal tool in achieving your weight loss goals.

My journey into the world of intermittent fasting was born not just out of professional interest, but also emotional necessity. Like many, I struggled with weight management for years, oscillating between diets that offered temporary benefits but never lasting change. It was during these years of trial and error that I stumbled upon the idea of intermittent energy restriction – a method that stood out due to its unique blend of simplicity and effectiveness.

The change I experienced was not just physical, but also mental and emotional. This was not just about shedding pounds; it was about getting a new perspective on health and nutrition. I felt compelled to share my results and experiences, leading to the birth of this book.

One of the fundamental aspects of successful weight loss that is often overlooked is knowing how our bodies work. Weight loss is not just about eating less and moving more; it's about knowing how our bodies respond to different foods, fasting, and various habits of eating.

In this book, we dig into how intermittent energy restriction helps in resetting your body's natural rhythms and metabolism. We explore the science behind why traditional diets often fail and how timed fasting can be a more effective method. This is not just a diet; it's a reorientation of how you see food, health, and your body.

By the end of this journey, you will not only have a deeper understanding of intermittent energy restriction but also a practical toolkit to apply it in your life. Whether you are new to the world of dieting or have been on this path for a while, this book is designed to provide insights and strategies that are both scientifically sound and practically doable.

Welcome to another section in your wellbeing process.Let's start on this enlightening path to a lighter, healthier you.

# Chapter 1

## The Core Concepts of Intermittent Energy Restriction

Intermittent energy restriction, often referred to as intermittent fasting (IF), is not a modern fad but a dietary approach deeply rooted in human history. At its core, IF includes cycling between periods of eating and fasting. It's a rhythmic approach to nutrition that fits with our evolutionary past.

The fasting periods in IF can run from a few hours to several days, but the most widely practiced forms involve daily fasting windows. For example, the 16/8 method involves fasting for 16 hours and eating during an 8-hour window.

## The Role of Ketosis

One of the key mechanisms behind IF is the induction of ketosis. When you fast, especially for long periods, your body depletes its glycogen stores, which are derived from carbohydrates. With limited glucose available for energy, your liver starts breaking down fat into molecules called ketones. Ketones can be used by cells as an additional fuel source.

This metabolic state, known as ketosis, is marked by increased fat burning. It's a key factor in the success of intermittent energy restriction for weight loss. By tapping into stored fat for energy, your body becomes a fat-burning machine during fasting times.

# Debunking Myths About Intermittent Fasting

**Myth 1:** Fasting Leads to Muscle Wasting

A common misconception about fasting is that it eventually leads to muscle loss. However, when done properly, IF can help preserve lean muscle mass. During fasting, your body prefers fat as an energy source while sparing protein and muscle tissue. This muscle-sparing effect is partly due to the increased production of growth hormone, which helps maintain lean body mass.

**Myth 2:** Fasting Slows Down Metabolism

Another myth is that fasting slows down metabolism, making it harder to lose weight. In fact, short-term fasting can temporarily boost metabolic rate. When you fast, your body becomes more efficient at burning calories for energy. This effect can continue even after you've broken your fast, resulting in increased calorie burn.

**Myth 3:** Fasting Causes Nutrient Deficiencies

Concerns about nutrient deficiencies are true, but intermittent energy restriction, when properly planned, doesn't necessarily lead to nutritional gaps. In fact, it can support a focus on nutrient-dense foods during eating windows. Moreover, supplements can help bridge any possible nutrient shortfalls. It's important to approach fasting with a balanced diet strategy.

**Fact 1:** Fasting Can Enhance Insulin Sensitivity

One of the scientifically confirmed benefits of intermittent fasting is its ability to improve insulin sensitivity. Insulin sensitivity is an important factor in managing blood sugar levels and preventing type 2 diabetes. When your body becomes more sensitive to insulin, it can regulate blood sugar more effectively, reducing the chance of insulin resistance and associated health issues.

**Fact 2:** Autophagy – The Cellular Cleaning Process

Intermittent fasting causes a fascinating process known as autophagy. Autophagy is the body's way of cleaning the house at the cellular level. During fasting, your cells go into repair mode, removing broken or dysfunctional components. This process plays a key role in maintaining cellular health and longevity.

**Fact 3:** Fasting Promotes Fat Adaptation
Intermittent fasting pushes the body to shift from relying on glucose (sugar) for energy to burning fat. This metabolic shift, known as fat adaptation, leads to better fat utilization and weight loss. It's a basic aspect of how intermittent energy restriction supports the reduction of body fat.

# The Hormonal Impact of Intermittent Fasting

Hormones play a key role in regulating metabolism and energy balance. Intermittent fasting has a profound impact on different hormones, contributing to its effectiveness in weight loss and overall health.

## Insulin: The Blood Sugar Regulator

Insulin is a hormone produced by the pancreas, and its main role is to regulate blood sugar levels. When you eat, especially carbohydrates, your blood sugar rises, causing the release of insulin. Insulin helps move glucose into cells for energy or storage.

During fasting periods in IF, insulin levels drop greatly. With fewer entering carbohydrates, there's less need for insulin. This drop in insulin levels is a key factor in increasing fat burning. When insulin is low, the body becomes more efficient at moving and utilizing stored fat for energy.

**Norepinephrine: The Metabolic Booster**

Norepinephrine, also known as noradrenaline, is a hormone and neurotransmitter that plays a part in the "fight or flight" response. It's released in reaction to stress and danger, but it also has metabolic effects.

Intermittent fasting can lead to higher norepinephrine production. This hormone helps improve metabolism and promote the breakdown of fat. It's part of the reason why fasting can lead to greater calorie burn and fat loss.

**Growth Hormone:** Preserving Lean Muscle Growth hormone (GH) is a hormone that causes growth and cell regeneration. It also plays a role in maintaining lean muscle mass. During fasting, GH levels tend to rise, helping to protect muscle tissue.

This preservation of muscle is important for overall body composition. It means that during fasting periods, your body mainly targets fat stores for energy, sparing precious muscle tissue. This is in opposition to some traditional diets that may lead to muscle loss along with fat loss.

## Creating a Caloric Deficit

Ultimately, intermittent fasting works on the principle of creating a caloric deficit. Weight loss happens when you consume fewer calories than you expend. IF achieves this by narrowing the window during which you eat, automatically reducing calorie intake.

By combining the metabolic advantages of fasting with calorie reduction, intermittent energy restriction offers an effective and sustainable approach to weight loss. It harnesses the body's natural ability to burn fat while giving flexibility in meal timing and food choices.

# Chapter 2

## The History of Fasting and Weight Loss

Fasting, as a dietary practice, has a history that goes back centuries and spans diverse cultures and civilizations. This chapter dives into the ancient wisdom that laid the foundation for the modern approach of intermittent energy restriction, highlighting the evolution of fasting diets through the ages.

## Ancient Wisdom

The Origins of Fasting

The idea of fasting for health and spiritual reasons can be traced to ancient civilizations. It was not simply a means of weight loss but a practice deeply intertwined with cultural, religious, and philosophical beliefs. Ancient Egyptians, Greeks, and Romans all adopted fasting into their rituals and healing practices.

## Egypt: The Practice of Therapeutic Fasting

In ancient Egypt, fasting was considered a healing practice. Medical papyri from around 1550 BCE documented fasting as a treatment for different ailments. Fasting was thought to purify the body and promote healing.

## Greece: Fasting in the Birthplace of Medicine

The Greeks, pioneers in the area of medicine, recognized the benefits of fasting. The famous physician Hippocrates, often referred to as the father of medicine, pushed for fasting to cleanse the body of toxins and promote overall health. His teachings laid the groundwork for the later growth of fasting as a medical practice.

## India: Fasting in Ayurveda

In India, the ancient method of Ayurveda includes fasting as a cleansing and healing practice. Fasting, known as "upavasa," is thought to purify the body and mind. It's often blended into Ayurvedic treatments to restore balance and vitality.

**Religious Fasting**

Many of the world's biggest religions incorporate fasting into their practices. In Christianity, Lent includes a period of fasting and reflection leading up to Easter. Muslims practice fasting during Ramadan as an act of devotion. Buddhism and Jainism also include fasting as part of their spiritual practice.

## Evolution of Fasting Diets Through the Ages

**The Middle Ages:**

During the Middle Ages, fasting took on a more pronounced religious importance. The Christian practice of fasting on designated days of the week or during specific seasons became widespread. Fasting was seen as a way to purify the soul and show devotion.

**The Renaissance: The Intersection of Art and Science**

The Renaissance age witnessed a resurgence of interest in science and human anatomy. Fasting was studied not only for its spiritual implications but also for its possible health benefits. Scholars like Leonardo da Vinci studied the effects of fasting on the human body, adding to a growing understanding of its physiological effects.

**The 19th Century: Fasting for Health**

The 19th century saw a return of interest in fasting as a therapeutic tool for health. Dr. John Harvey Kellogg, a famous figure in the development of breakfast cereals, advocated for fasting as a means to cleanse the body and prevent illness. He even ran sanitariums where fasting was a central component of treatment.

## The Early 20th Century: Fasting and the Fasting Movement

Fasting got momentum in the early 20th century, with notable figures like Dr. Otto Buchinger and Arnold Ehret championing its health benefits. Fasting clinics and sanitariums expanded, offering supervised fasting programs. Fasting was touted as a way to treat a range of conditions, from obesity to digestive disorders.

## The Mid-20th Century: Scientific Exploration

As science and medicine advanced, researchers began to examine fasting's physiological effects more rigorously. Studies explored fasting's effect on metabolism, insulin sensitivity, and weight loss. Fasting was no longer just a fringe practice but a subject of scientific study.

## The Late 20th Century: The Advent of Intermittent Fasting

The late 20th century saw the emergence of intermittent fasting as a structured method to fasting. Dr. Michael Mosley's 5:2 diet, which involves eating normally for five days and greatly reducing calorie intake for two non-consecutive days, gained popularity. This marked a shift from prolonged fasting to more manageable and sustainable fasting practices.

## The 21st Century: Intermittent Energy Restriction

In the 21st century, intermittent energy restriction has become a focal point of study and a popular method for weight management and overall health. The idea of fasting windows, such as the 16/8 method (fasting for 16 hours and eating during an 8-hour window), gained widespread attention.

## The Modern Approach to Fasting

Today, intermittent energy restriction represents a fusion of ancient wisdom, historical practices, and current science understanding. It recognises the profound effects of fasting on metabolism, insulin sensitivity, and fat adaptation, while also emphasizing sustainability and flexibility.

Intermittent energy restriction understands that fasting need not be an all-or-nothing approach. It helps people to tailor fasting patterns to their lifestyles and preferences. This adaptability has added to its popularity and effectiveness in the modern era.

In summary, the past of fasting and weight loss is a journey that spans millennia. From its beginnings in ancient societies and religious traditions to its evolution into a structured and scientifically studied approach, fasting has endured and adapted. It continues to offer important insights into health, wellness, and the human relationship with food.

# Chapter 3

## Crafting Your Personal Fasting Plan

As you embark on your journey of intermittent energy restriction, it's important to craft a fasting plan that aligns with your goals, lifestyle, and preferences. This chapter covers the different types of intermittent fasting, helping you find the right fit for you. Additionally, we'll delve into the art of building a sustainable fasting schedule that ensures long-term success.

## Types of Intermittent Fasting: Finding Your Fit

Intermittent fasting is not a one-size-fits-all method. It offers a range of fasting patterns, allowing you to choose the one that suits your needs and fits with your daily routine. Let's explore some of the most famous types of intermittent fasting:

## 1. The 16/8 Method

The 16/8 method is one of the simplest and most widely practiced kinds of intermittent fasting. It includes fasting for 16 hours and eating during an 8-hour window. For example, you might skip breakfast and eat your first meal at noon, finishing your last meal by 8 PM. .

## 2. The 5:2 Diet

The 5:2 diet, popularized by Dr. Michael Mosley, consists of eating normally for five days of the week and greatly reducing calorie intake (around 500-600 calories) for two non-consecutive days. These fasting days can be picked to fit your schedule. It offers flexibility while still offering the benefits of intermittent fasting.

## 3. **Eat-Stop-Eat**

This technique includes fasting for an entire 24 hours more than once per week. For example, you might fast from dinner one day to dinner the next day. This approach can be challenging for beginners but can be highly effective for weight loss and fat burning when done properly.

## 4. **The Warrior Diet**

The Warrior Diet involves fasting for 20 hours and eating within a 4-hour window in the evening. During the fasting time, you can consume small amounts of raw fruits and vegetables or light snacks. This approach is inspired by the eating habits of ancient warriors and aligns with the concept of undereating during the day and feasting in the evening.

## 5. Alternate-Day Fasting

Alternate-day fasting alternates between days of normal eating and days of fasting or consuming very few calories (around 500-600 calories). It offers a clear structure but can be more challenging due to the alternating nature of the fasting days.

## 6. OMAD (One Meal a Day)

OMAD means fasting for 23 hours and consuming all your daily calories in a single meal. This method is highly restrictive in terms of meal timing but allows for flexibility in food choices during the one meal.

## Creating a Sustainable Fasting Schedule

### Listen to Your Body

When crafting your fasting plan, it's crucial to listen to your body's signals and change accordingly. Not every fasting method will suit everyone, and it's important to be attuned to how your body responds. If a particular fasting pattern causes excessive hunger, fatigue, or discomfort, consider trying a different method.

### Gradual Transition

If you're new to intermittent fasting, consider a gradual shift. Start with a shorter fasting window, such as 12 hours, and gradually lengthen it as your body adapts. This can make the adjustment process easier and more sustainable.

## Meal Timing Matters

The timing of your meals within the eating window can affect your fasting experience. It's a good practice to have a balanced meal that includes protein, healthy fats, and fiber to help keep you satiated during the fasting time. Experiment with different meal times to see what works best for your energy levels and hunger cues.

## Stay Hydrated

During fasting periods, it's important to stay hydrated. Water, herbal teas, and black coffee (without added sugar or cream) are usually allowed during fasting. Proper hydration can help manage hunger and support general well-being.

**Flexibility Is Key**

Intermittent fasting is not about strict rules but about flexibility and sustainability. It should improve your life, not disrupt it. If a social event or special occasion falls outside your fasting schedule, it's okay to change your plan for that day and resume your fasting routine afterward. The key is long-term stability, not perfection.

**Consult a Healthcare Professional**

Before embarking on any fasting regimen, especially if you have underlying health conditions, it's advisable to visit a healthcare professional. They can provide guidance tailored to your individual needs and ensure that fasting is safe and suitable for you.

Crafting your personal fasting plan is an exciting step towards meeting your health and weight loss goals. It includes selecting the intermittent fasting method that resonates with you and aligns with your daily life. Remember that there's no one-size-fits-all approach, and it's okay to try to find what works best for you.

# Chapter 4

## Nutrition and Fasting – The Perfect Pair

Intermittent fasting and nutrition are two sides of the same coin when it comes to improving your health and well-being. This chapter dives into the symbiotic relationship between nutrition and fasting, stressing how they complement each other to create a powerful foundation for a healthier lifestyle.

### Understanding the Fusion of Nutrition and Fasting

Intermittent eating is not solely about when you eat; it's equally concerned with what you eat. Nutrition plays a pivotal role in maximizing the benefits of fasting and ensuring your body gets the essential nutrients it needs to thrive.

## 1. Synergy of Weight Management

Fasting periods cause a caloric deficit, contributing to weight loss. However, what you eat during non-fasting periods can affect the quality of this weight loss. Opting for nutrient-dense foods ensures that your body gets the important vitamins, minerals, and antioxidants it needs while shedding excess pounds.

## 2. Enhancing Metabolic Health

Intermittent fasting has been linked to improved metabolic health, including better insulin sensitivity and blood sugar control. Complementing fasting with a balanced diet further supports these metabolic effects.

Foods rich in fiber, lean proteins, and healthy fats support stable blood sugar levels and efficient metabolism.

### 3. **Promoting Cellular Health**

Fasting causes autophagy, a cellular cleaning process that removes damaged components and supports cellular health. Proper nutrition gives the building blocks for cellular repair and regeneration. Ensuring you consume important nutrients like amino acids, antioxidants, and omega-3 fatty acids can amplify the cellular benefits of fasting.

# Eating Right During Non-Fasting Periods

While fasting periods are characterized by abstaining from food, non-fasting periods provide a chance to nourish your body with wholesome foods. Let's discuss some principles of eating right during these windows:

## 1. Focus on Entire Food varieties

Entire food varieties, like natural products, vegetables, entire grains, lean proteins, and sound fats, ought to frame the premise of your eating regimen. These food sources are wealthy in supplements and give supported energy, pursuing them a magnificent decision for non-fasting times.

## 2. Adjusted Feasts

Make adjusted feasts that incorporate a blend of macronutrients: carbs, proteins, and fats. This equilibrium keeps up with glucose levels, advances satiety, and gives a consistent wellspring of energy.

## 3. Careful Eating

Practice careful eating by partaking in each nibble, focusing on appetite and totality signals, and keeping away from interruptions while eating. Care makes a better relationship with food and can forestall gorging.

## 4. Hydration

Remain hydrated over the course of the day by drinking water, home grown teas, and other non-caloric fluids. Satisfactory hydration upholds processing, digestion, and general prosperity.

## 5. **Fiber-Rich Food varieties**

Consolidate fiber-rich food varieties like natural products, veggies, and entire grains into your dinners. Fiber helps processing, helps keep a solid weight, and supports stomach wellbeing.

## 6. **Lean Proteins**

Include lean forms of protein such as poultry, fish, tofu, and legumes in your diet. Protein is important for muscle maintenance, immune function, and overall health.

## 7. **Healthy Fats**

Choose healthy fats like bananas, nuts, seeds, and olive oil. These fats provide important fatty acids and support brain health, heart health, and satiety.

## 8. Limit Processed Foods

Minimize processed and ultra-processed foods that are high in added sugars, unhealthy fats, and fake additives. These foods can disrupt your metabolic health and should be eaten sparingly.

## 9. Balanced Snacking

If you choose to snack during non-fasting times, opt for balanced snacks that combine protein, fiber, and healthy fats. Examples include Greek yogurt with berries or a small amount of nuts.

10. **Adapt to Your Lifestyle**

Tailor your eating patterns to your lifestyle and tastes. Intermittent fasting allows flexibility in meal timing, so choose a schedule that fits with your daily routine.

## Essential Nutrients for Optimal Health

Optimal nutrition during non-fasting periods includes ensuring you receive essential nutrients that support overall health and well-being. Let's study some of these key nutrients:

### 1. Vitamins and Minerals

A diverse diet rich in fruits and vegetables offers a broad spectrum of vitamins and minerals. Vitamins like vitamin C, vitamin

D, and vitamin K, as well as minerals like calcium, magnesium, and potassium, play vital roles in different bodily functions.

## 2. Omega-3 Fatty Acids

Omega-3 fatty acids, found in fatty fish like salmon and flaxseeds, offer anti-inflammatory effects and support heart and brain health.

## 3. Protein

Protein is important for muscle maintenance, immune function, and the production of enzymes and hormones. Incorporate lean amounts of protein into your meals.

## 4. Fiber

Fiber aids digestion, promotes feelings of fullness, and supports gut health. Whole grains, fruits, and vegetables are great sources of dietary fiber.

## 5. Antioxidants

Antioxidants like vitamin C, vitamin E, and beta-carotene help combat oxidative stress and reduce the chance of chronic diseases.

## 7. Calcium and Vitamin D

Calcium and vitamin D are important for bone health. Dairy products, leafy greens, and fortified foods can help meet these nutrition needs.

# Chapter 5

## Fasting, Exercise, and Lifcstyle

Integrating intermittent fasting into your life involves more than just adjusting your eating habits. This chapter explores the dynamic relationship between fasting, exercise, and lifestyle adjustments, giving insights into how they can work together to improve your health and well-being.

## Balancing Exercise with Fasting

Exercise and intermittent fasting can be strong allies in your quest for better health and vitality. However, achieving the right balance between the two is important for a successful fasting journey.

## 1. Timing Matters

When you exercise during your fasting periods, it's important to consider timing. Exercising in a fasted state, such as in the morning before your first meal, can increase fat burning. Fasting primes your body to use saved fat for energy during workouts. However, intense or prolonged workouts may be more difficult in a fasted state, so it's important to listen to your body.

## 2. Moderate Intensity

Moderate-intensity workouts, such as brisk walking, jogging, or yoga, are well-suited for fasting times. They provide the benefits of exercise without overly taxing your energy stores. High-intensity workouts or prolonged endurance exercises may be better suited for non-fasting times when you can refuel after the session.

## 3. Post-Workout Nutrition

After a workout, whether in a fasting or non-fasting state, favor post-workout nutrition. Consuming a balanced meal or snack that includes protein and carbohydrates can support muscle recovery and refill glycogen stores.

## 4. Adaptation Over Time

Your body will adapt to exercise and fasting habits over time. As you become more accustomed to intermittent fasting, you may find that your energy levels and exercise ability improve during fasting times. It's important to be patient with yourself as you navigate these adaptations.

5. **Variety Is Key**

Incorporate a range of exercise modalities into your routine. Include strength training, cardiovascular workouts, and flexibility exercises to ensure a well-rounded fitness routine. Mixing up your workouts can also avoid boredom and plateaus.

## Lifestyle Adjustments for Better Results

Intermittent fasting is not a standalone practice but a part of your wider lifestyle. Making thoughtful adjustments to various parts of your life can enhance the results you achieve with fasting.

## 1. **Sleep and Recovery**

Adequate sleep and recovery are important for overall well-being and the success of your fasting journey. Prioritize excellent sleep to support hormonal balance and optimize the benefits of fasting. Create a sleep-friendly environment and create a consistent sleep schedule.

## 2. **Stress Management**

Chronic stress can disrupt hormonal balance and affect fasting findings. Implement stress management methods such as meditation, deep breathing exercises, or mindfulness to reduce stress levels. A balanced lifestyle that includes relaxation and leisure activities can also help to overall well-being.

### 3. Time Management

Efficient time management can help you stick to your fasting schedule and make healthier choices. Plan your meals and tasks in advance to reduce decision fatigue and prevent impulsive eating. Use tools like meal prep and time-blocking to improve your day.

### 4. Mindful Eating

Practicing mindful eating goes beyond mealtimes. It includes cultivating awareness of your eating habits and the choices you make. Be mindful of portion sizes, food decisions, and the emotional aspects of eating. Mindful eating can help avoid overeating and support your fasting goals.

## 5. **Professional Guidance**

Consider consulting with healthcare workers, registered dietitians, or fitness experts for personalized advice. They can assess your specific needs, provide tailored suggestions, and ensure that fasting aligns with your health and wellness goals.

## 6. **Long-Term Sustainability**

Intermittent fasting is a lifestyle method, not a short-term fix. Focus on long-term sustainability by making gradual changes that fit with your preferences and values. Sustainable changes are more likely to yield lasting effects.

## 7. **Self-Care**

Prioritize self-care and self-compassion throughout your fasting journey. Engage in activities that bring you joy and relaxation, whether it's reading, sports, or spending time with loved ones.

In conclusion, balancing exercise with fasting and making thoughtful lifestyle adjustments are integral aspects of a successful intermittent fasting path. By considering the time of your workouts, maintaining hydration, and adapting your exercise routine, you can maximize the benefits of both fasting and physical activity. Lifestyle adjustments, including stress management, sleep prioritization, and mindful eating, can further enhance your fasting experience and general well-being.

# Chapter 6

## Overcoming Challenges and Plateaus

While intermittent fasting offers numerous benefits, it's not without its challenges and possible plateaus. This chapter addresses these hurdles and offers effective strategies for breaking through weight loss plateaus, ensuring you can continue on your path to better health.

## Common Hurdles in Intermittent Fasting

Intermittent fasting, like any lifestyle change, comes with its set of common challenges that people may face on their journey. Recognizing these hurdles is the first step toward beating them.

## 1. Hunger Pangs and Cravings

Hunger pangs and cravings, especially during fasting times, can be challenging to manage. The sensation of hunger is normal and can be a sign that your body is adjusting to a new eating routine. To fight this, drink water, herbal tea, or black coffee to help curb your appetite. You can also try distracting yourself with light activities or mindfulness techniques to redirect your attention.

## 2. Social Pressures

Social situations, gatherings, or peer pressure to eat outside your fasting window can be challenging to manage. It's important to communicate your fasting goals with friends and family to gain their support. You can also plan ahead by eating before social events or bringing fasting-friendly snacks to avoid feeling left out.

## 3. Energy Levels

Some individuals may experience fluctuations in energy levels during fasting, especially when first starting. This can affect daily tasks and exercise routines. To address this, ensure you're getting adequate rest, staying hydrated, and consuming balanced meals during non-fasting times. As your body changes to fasting, your energy levels may become more stable.

## 4. Plateaus in Weight Loss

Weight loss plateaus are a regular concern for individuals on an intermittent fasting journey. After initial success, it's possible to reach a point where weight loss stalls. Plateaus can be frustrating, but they're not unusual. Understanding the causes and tactics to break through them can be empowering.

## Strategies to Break Through Weight Loss Plateaus

When you encounter a weight loss plateau in your intermittent fasting journey, it's important to remain patient and persistent. Here are techniques to help you overcome plateaus and continue progressing toward your goals:

1. **Review Your Eating Habits**

Take a close look at your dietary choices during non-fasting times. Are you consuming nutrient-dense foods, balancing macronutrients, and practicing thoughtful eating? Sometimes, making small changes to your diet can reignite weight loss progress.

## 2. Adjust Your Fasting Window

Consider modifying your fasting time. Experiment with different fasting durations or schedules to see if your body acts differently. You might lengthen or shorten fasting periods or change the time of day when you break your fast.

## 3. Incorporate Exercise

Regular physical activity can support weight loss attempts and help break through plateaus. Incorporate a mix of cardio and strength training routines into your routine. Exercise can improve metabolism, increase muscle mass, and enhance fat burning.

## 4. Track Your Progress

Maintain a detailed record of your meals, fasting times, exercise routines, and how you feel physically and emotionally. Tracking your success can provide insights into what's working and where adjustments are needed.

## 5. Manage Stress

Chronic stress can hinder weight loss and lead to plateaus. Prioritize stress management methods like meditation, deep breathing, or yoga. Reducing stress levels can positively impact endocrine balance and metabolism.

## 6. Stay Hydrated

Proper hydration is important for overall well-being and can support weight loss. Drinking enough water can help control appetite, improve digestion, and optimize metabolic processes.

## 7. Get Adequate Sleep

Quality sleep is important for weight management and overall health. Aim for 7-9 hours of sleep per night. Sleep deprivation can upset hormonal balance, making it harder to lose weight.

## 8. Reevaluate Your Goals

Sometimes, weight loss plateaus appear because your body has reached a healthy set point. Reevaluate your goals and consider whether weight loss is still the main focus or if other health improvements, such as increased energy or better metabolic health, are equally valuable.

## 9. Consider Intermittent Fasting Variations

If you've been following a specific intermittent fasting method, consider variations. Different fasting regimes, such as alternate-day fasting or the 5:2 diet, might provide a new stimulus for weight loss.

## 10. Seek Support

Engage with a supportive community or seek advice from a healthcare professional or registered dietitian. They can provide personalized advice, spot potential barriers, and offer solutions tailored to your unique needs.

## 11. **Be Patient and Persistent**

Breaking through a weight loss rut may take time. Remember that plateaus are a normal part of the journey, and consistency is key.

## Celebrate Non-Scale Victories

While the scale is one way to measure progress, it's important to celebrate non-scale victories as well. These victories include improved energy levels, better sleep, enhanced mood, and increased general well-being. Recognizing these successes can provide motivation and keep you focused on your health journey's holistic benefits.

Overcoming challenges and plateaus in intermittent fasting takes a combination of strategies, patience, and perseverance. By understanding common hurdles and implementing effective techniques to break through plateaus, you can continue on your road to better health and well-being.

# Chapter 7

## Beyond Weight Loss - Other Health Benefits

Intermittent fasting is praised not only for its role in weight management but also for its potential to improve overall health and well-being. This chapter explores the myriad health benefits of intermittent fasting beyond weight loss, stressing its role in longevity, disease prevention, and mental and emotional well-being.

## Fasting for Longevity and Disease Prevention

Unlocking the Secrets of Longevity
Throughout history, people have sought the fountain of youth, and while no such magical fountain exists, intermittent fasting

has emerged as a promising method for promoting longevity. Research on various organisms, from yeast to mammals, has shown that fasting can trigger cellular processes that increase longevity.

One of the key processes at play is autophagy, the cellular self-cleaning process. During fasting, when the body experiences a break from constant digestion, it changes its focus to repair and recycling. Autophagy becomes more active, clearing out damaged cellular components and adding to cellular rejuvenation.

Caloric restriction, a practice closely linked to fasting, has also been associated with increased lifespan in various studies. Fasting mimics some of the effects of caloric restriction, such as reduced insulin levels, improved insulin sensitivity, and a decrease in inflammation, all of which are linked to longevity.

## Disease Prevention through Fasting

Intermittent fasting demonstrates considerable potential in the prevention of different chronic diseases, including:

1. Type 2 Diabetes: Fasting can improve insulin sensitivity, regulate blood sugar levels, and lower the risk of type 2 diabetes. It helps the body to reset its insulin response and improve glucose metabolism.

2. Heart Disease: Fasting can lead to reductions in risk factors for heart disease, such as high blood pressure, inflammation,

and high amounts of triglycerides. It also helps heart health by promoting weight loss and improving cholesterol profiles.

3. Neurodegenerative Diseases: Emerging research shows that fasting may have neuroprotective effects. It can activate pathways that enhance brain health and reduce the chance of neurodegenerative conditions like Alzheimer's and Parkinson's disease.

4. Cancer: Fasting may affect cancer prevention by reducing the chance of tumor formation and supporting the body's natural defense mechanisms. It can also improve the effectiveness of cancer treatments.

5. Inflammation: Chronic inflammation is a root cause of many illnesses. Fasting can reduce inflammation markers in the body, adding to the prevention of inflammatory diseases.

6. Age-Related Conditions: Intermittent fasting has been linked with a decreased risk of age-related conditions, including sarcopenia (muscle loss), osteoporosis (bone loss), and frailty.

## The Role of Cellular Health

At the cellular level, fasting's impact on disease prevention and longevity can be attributed to several factors:

1. Enhanced Autophagy: As stated earlier, autophagy plays a crucial role in cellular

health. By clearing out damaged components and supporting cellular repair, fasting adds to the overall well-being of cells.

2. Reduced Oxidative Stress: Fasting lowers oxidative stress on cells, preventing damage caused by free radicals. This oxidative stress reduction is linked to a lower chance of chronic diseases.

3. Improved Insulin Sensitivity: Fasting improves insulin sensitivity, making cells more responsive to insulin. This, in turn, helps regulate blood sugar levels and lowers the risk of type 2 diabetes.

4. Hormonal Balance: Fasting can affect the balance of hormones like insulin, human

growth hormone (HGH), and cortisol, all of which play critical roles in aging, metabolism, and disease prevention.

## Mental and Emotional Benefits of Intermittent Fasting

**Cognitive Clarity and Focus**

Intermittent fasting has been linked with better cognitive function and mental clarity. During fasting times, the body switches to burning ketones (derived from fat) for energy instead of glucose. This shift in energy source can improve mental focus and cognitive function.

Additionally, fasting supports brain health by promoting the production of brain-derived neurotrophic factor (BDNF), a protein that supports the growth and repair of brain cells. Higher BDNF levels are linked with better cognitive function and reduced chance of neurodegenerative diseases.

**Emotional Well-Being**

Intermittent fasting can have good benefits on emotional well-being and mood regulation. It's thought that fasting helps regulate the production of neurotransmitters like serotonin, which plays a crucial role in mood stabilization. Some individuals report feeling more balanced emotionally and having reduced mood swings while practicing intermittent fasting.

Furthermore, fasting may support mental resilience by enhancing stress responses and reducing cortisol levels. Chronic stress is a major contributor to mood disorders, and fasting's stress-reducing benefits can have a profound impact on emotional well-being.

**Increased Energy Levels**

Many people who follow intermittent fasting report increased energy levels and improved overall vitality. This boost in energy can add to a more positive outlook on life and a greater capacity for physical and mental activities.

**Mental Resilience**

Intermittent fasting fosters mental resilience and self-discipline. Successfully adhering to a fasting schedule requires planning, self-control, and dedication. Over time, these qualities can spill over into other areas of life, leading to greater self-confidence and personal growth.

## The Gut-Brain Connection

Emerging research shows a strong connection between gut health and mental well-being. Intermittent fasting may positively influence the gut microbiome, supporting a balanced and diverse community of beneficial bacteria. A healthy gut microbiome is linked with better mood, reduced anxiety, and enhanced mental health.

# Chapter 8

## Preparing for Long-Term Success

As you embark on your intermittent fasting journey, it's important to plan for long-term success. This chapter focuses on strategies for staying motivated, tracking your progress successfully, and adjusting your fasting plan to accommodate life changes. By preparing for the long haul, you can ensure that intermittent fasting stays a sustainable and rewarding lifestyle choice.

# Staying Motivated and Tracking Progress

## Setting and Revisiting Goals

Motivation is the driving force behind any great journey. Start by setting clear and realistic goals for your intermittent fasting journey. These goals can be linked to weight loss, improved health markers, or other personal objectives. Having specific goals provides you with a sense of purpose and direction.

However, goals aren't set. It's important to revisit and adjust them as needed. Celebrate your successes, whether they are small milestones or major achievements. Recognize the work you've made and use that momentum to keep moving forward.

**Creating a Visual Timeline**

A visual timeline can be a powerful motivating tool. Create a calendar or chart that shows your fasting schedule, goals, and progress. Use colors, stickers, or other visual cues to mark fasting days, successful adherence, and milestones met. Seeing your journey laid out can reinforce your commitment and inspire you to stay on track.

**Building a Support System**

Intermittent fasting can be a solitary activity, but it doesn't have to be. Building a support system can significantly impact your drive and success. Share your goals with friends, family members, or a fasting group. Having people who understand and support your journey can provide encouragement, responsibility, and a sense of belonging.

**Daily Affirmations and Mindset**

A positive attitude is a crucial component of long-term success. Incorporate daily affirmations or motivational quotes into your practice. These can serve as memories of your commitment and help you stay focused on your goals. Cultivating a growth mindset, where setbacks are viewed as opportunities for learning and growth, can also improve resilience and motivation.

## Tracking Your Progress

Effective progress tracking allows you to gauge the effect of intermittent fasting on your health and well-being. Consider the following tracking methods:

1. Food Journal

Keeping a food journal can help you monitor your eating habits, track calorie intake, and identify areas for growth. Record what you eat, when you eat, and how you feel during and after eating.

2. Body Measurements:

In addition to weighing yourself, measure key body markers such as waist circumference, hip circumference, and body fat percentage. Changes in these measurements can provide a more complete view of your progress.

3. Health Markers:

If you have specific health goals, work with your healthcare provider to monitor important health markers, such as blood pressure, cholesterol levels, and blood sugar levels. Improvements in these markers can be motivating and indicative of better health.

4. Fitness Levels:

Track your fitness growth by recording exercise routines, strength gains, and endurance improvements. Regular exercise can complement your fasting journey and add to overall well-being.

5. Mood and Energy:

Keep a record of your mood, energy levels, and mental clarity. Note any changes you feel as you continue intermittent fasting. Improved mood and greater energy can be powerful motivators.

**Celebrating Non-Scale Victories**

While weight reduction might be an essential objective, it's critical to celebrate non-scale triumphs too. These wins encompass improvements in health markers, increased energy levels, better sleep, enhanced mood, and greater overall well-being. Recognizing and celebrating these successes can provide motivation, even if the scale doesn't always reflect your progress.

**Periodic Assessments**

Set aside regular intervals for thorough assessments of your fasting journey. These assessments can include reviewing your goals, tracking success, and evaluating any challenges or adjustments needed. By regularly assessing your journey, you can make informed choices about your fasting plan and stay motivated over the long term.

## Adjusting Your Plan for Life Changes

### Adapting to Life Events

Life is dynamic, and unexpected events can affect your fasting routine. Whether it's holidays, vacations, work duties, or family changes, there will be times when adjustments are necessary. Rather than viewing these events as obstacles, see them as chances to practice flexibility and adaptability.

## Creating a Fasting Toolbox

Develop a toolbox of fasting tactics that you can draw upon when life changes occur. This toolbox can include:

Fasting Variations:

Explore different fasting methods, such as time-restricted eating, alternate-day fasting, or the 5:2 diet. Having multiple approaches in your toolbox allows you to choose the one that best fits your current circumstances.

Meal Planning:

Learn how to plan meals that fit with your fasting schedule. Meal prep and planning can help you stay on track, even during busy times.

Intermittent Fasting Apps:
Use fasting apps or digital tools to automate and track your fasting routine. These apps can provide reminders, tracking, and help.

Mindfulness and Stress Management: Practice mindfulness and stress-reduction techniques to help you stay grounded and make mindful food choices, even in challenging conditions.

## Seeking Professional Guidance

If you encounter major life changes, consider consulting with a healthcare provider or registered dietitian. They can provide guidance on adjusting your fasting plan to accommodate your unique wants and circumstances. Professional support can be invaluable in ensuring that intermittent fasting stays a sustainable and health-promoting practice.

Preparing for long-term success in intermittent fasting requires a mix of motivation, progress tracking, and adaptability. By setting and revisiting goals, building a support system, and tracking your progress effectively, you can stay motivated throughout your trip. Additionally, by developing strategies for adapting to life changes and seeking professional advice when needed, you can ensure that intermittent fasting remains a sustainable and satisfying lifestyle choice.

# Chapter 9

## Success Stories and Case Studies

In this chapter, the real-life success stories and case studies of people who have embraced intermittent fasting as a lifestyle. By examining these stories, we gain insights into the transformative power of intermittent fasting and the important lessons learned from both successes and failures.

### Real-Life Transformations

Sarah's Journey to Health and Wellness

Sarah, a 38-year-old marketing executive and mother of two, battled with weight gain and low energy for years. She felt trapped in a cycle of fad diets that gave short-term results but left her feeling deprived and unsatisfied. Sarah chose to explore intermittent fasting as a more sustainable approach.

Sarah's journey began with a 16:8 fasting plan, which involved fasting for 16 hours and eating within an 8-hour window. Initially, she found it challenging to change to this new eating pattern, but with time, it became a natural part of her routine.

Over the course of several months, Sarah experienced major changes. She lost weight, her energy levels soared, and her mood improved. What made intermittent fasting different for Sarah was the freedom it offered. She could enjoy meals with her family without feeling guilty, and the lack of constant food focus gave her mental clarity and freedom.

Sarah's transformation went beyond weight loss. Her blood pressure and cholesterol numbers improved, and she felt more in control of her health. Sarah's success story shows the long-term sustainability of intermittent fasting as a lifestyle choice.

Lessons from Sarah's Success: Flexibility Is Key: Intermittent fasting allowed Sarah to enjoy both her family meals and the perks of fasting. Flexibility is a key factor in making fasting sustainable.

Mental Clarity: Sarah experienced better mental clarity and focus. Intermittent fasting can improve cognitive function, which is often overlooked.

Health Improvements: Beyond weight loss, Sarah saw improvements in her blood pressure and cholesterol levels, emphasizing the wider health benefits of fasting.

John's Journey: A Lesson from Setbacks
John, a 45-year-old IT worker, was inspired by the success stories of intermittent fasting. Eager to achieve similar results, he began an aggressive fasting regimen without proper direction. John attempted a prolonged water fast, hoping for rapid weight loss.

However, John's approach proved unsustainable and possibly harmful. He suffered severe fatigue, dizziness, and muscle weakness. Concerned for his health, John contacted a healthcare provider, who advised him to discontinue the extreme fasting and adopt a more balanced approach.

John's experience shows the importance of seeking professional guidance and gradual progress when incorporating intermittent fasting into one's lifestyle.

Lessons from John's Setback:
Gradual Progress: Intermittent fasting should be tackled gradually, especially for those new to fasting. Extreme fasting can have harmful effects on health.

Professional Guidance: Consulting with a healthcare provider or certified dietitian is crucial to ensure that fasting is safe and appropriate for individual circumstances.

Lessons from Successes and Failures

Intermittent fasting is a powerful tool, but it's important to approach it with a balanced and informed perspective. The success stories of individuals like Sarah show the transformative potential of fasting when applied thoughtfully and sustainably.

Conversely, John's experience underscores the importance of avoiding extreme fasting practices and seeking professional advice to ensure safety and efficacy.

Key Takeaways:

Sustainability: Intermittent fasting is most successful when it becomes a sustainable living choice rather than a short-term diet.

Flexibility: Fasting offers flexibility, allowing individuals to enjoy meals with loved ones and keep a balanced relationship with food.

Gradual Progress: Newcomers to intermittent fasting should start gradually and avoid extreme fasting practices.

Professional Guidance: Seeking guidance from healthcare providers or registered dietitians is important, especially when dealing with health conditions or planning major dietary changes.

Health Benefits: Intermittent fasting offers a range of health benefits beyond weight loss, including improved cognitive function, better mood, and enhanced overall well-being.

Real-life success stories and case studies provide valuable insights into the transformative possibilities of intermittent fasting. By learning from both successes and setbacks, individuals can approach fasting with a balanced and informed viewpoint. The key to long-term success lies in sustainability, flexibility, gradual progress, and, when needed, seeking professional advice.

# Conclusion

## Your New Lifestyle Awaits

As we end this journey through the world of intermittent fasting, you stand on the threshold of a new and empowered lifestyle. The insights, strategies, and real-life stories shared in this book have equipped you with the knowledge and tools needed to start on a transformative journey toward health and wellness. In this final chapter, we'll reflect on the key takeaways and provide advice on embracing the fasting lifestyle.

Key Takeaways

1. Intermittent Fasting Is a Lifestyle, Not a Diet

Understanding that intermittent fasting is a sustainable lifestyle choice is essential. Unlike restrictive diets, intermittent fasting offers flexibility and adaptability, making it a lifelong pledge to your health and well-being.

2. Sustainability Is the Cornerstone

Sustainability is the cornerstone of intermittent fasting success. Whether you choose time-restricted eating, alternate-day fasting, or another approach, your fasting regimen should be something you can comfortably integrate into your life for the long run.

3. Gradual Progress Yields Lasting Results

Avoid the urge to rush into extreme fasting practices. Gradual progress helps your body to adapt and minimizes the risk of adverse effects. Small, sustainable changes lead to lasting effects.

4. Flexibility and Freedom

Intermittent fasting offers flexibility and freedom in your eating patterns. You can enjoy meals with loved ones, savor your favorite foods, and still reap the benefits of fasting. It's a mindset that aligns with your life rather than disrupts it.

5. Professional Guidance Matters

If you have specific health concerns, it's wise to seek professional advice. Healthcare providers and registered dietitians can give personalized recommendations and ensure that intermittent fasting is safe and appropriate for your circumstances.

## Embracing the Fasting Lifestyle

1. Set Clear and Achievable Goals

As you continue your fasting journey, set clear and realistic goals. These goals will provide you with direction and drive. Praise your triumphs en route, regardless of how little they might appear.

2. Build a Support System

Surround yourself with a support system of friends, family, or like-minded people who understand and encourage your fasting journey. Share your experiences, seek advice, and give support to others on similar paths.

## 3. Track Your Progress

Effective progress tracking is important. Keep a food journal, measure body metrics, watch health markers, and assess your mental and emotional well-being. Tracking allows you to gauge the impact of fasting on your health and offers motivation.

## 4. Embrace Flexibility

Life is dynamic, and changes are expected. Embrace the freedom that intermittent fasting offers. Learn to adapt your fasting plan to suit life events, vacations, celebrations, and unforeseen circumstances.

5. Celebrate Non-Scale Victories

While weight loss may be a main goal, don't overlook non-scale victories. Celebrate improvements in your health markers, energy levels, mood, and general well-being. These victories are equally important.

6. Practice Mindfulness and Self-Compassion

Mindfulness and self-compassion are strong tools in your fasting journey. Be caring to yourself, particularly during testing times. Practice care to settle on careful food choices and develop a positive association with food.

7. Share Your Journey

As you experience the benefits of intermittent fasting, consider sharing your journey with others. Your success story may inspire and support others who are seeking good changes in their lives. Be a source of encouragement and strength.

Your journey to health and wellness is a lifelong goal. Intermittent fasting has given you a valuable tool and a sustainable lifestyle choice. As you move forward, understand that your path is unique, and your goals are personal. Embrace the fasting lifestyle with excitement and openness.

As you take the final steps of this book's journey, do so with confidence and a deep-seated belief in your ability to create a healthier, more lively future for yourself. Your journey may have started with curiosity, but it now continues with purpose and drive.

As we bid farewell to this book, we offer our best wishes for your continued success and well-being. May your fasting lifestyle bring you the health, energy, and happiness you seek. Remember that the journey is as rewarding as the goal, and your commitment to a healthier you is a journey worth taking.

Thank you for allowing us to be part of your fasting journey. Farewell, and may your future be filled with health, wellness, and the fulfillment of your goals.

# Appendix: Resources and Recipes

In this comprehensive appendix, you'll find a wealth of tools and valuable information to support your intermittent fasting journey. From delicious fasting-friendly recipes to scientific studies and literature, this appendix serves as a useful reference for your continued success.

## Fasting-Friendly Recipes

### Breakfast Delights

 Berry Blast Smoothie Ingredients:

1/2 cup of mixed berries (strawberries, blueberries, raspberries)

1/2 ripe banana

1/2 cup Greek yogurt

1 tablespoon honey (optional)

Ice cubes (optional)


Instructions: Blend all the items until smooth.

Pour into a glass and enjoy a refreshing and antioxidant-rich breakfast drink.


Veggie Omelette Ingredients:

2 eggs

1/4 cup chopped bell peppers (red, green, and yellow)

1/4 cup diced tomatoes

1/4 cup diced onions

Salt and pepper to taste


Directions: In a bowl, beat the eggs and season with salt and pepper.

Heat a non-stick skillet over medium heat and add the diced veggies.

Pour the beaten eggs over the veggies and cook until the edges start to set.

Carefully fold the omelette in half and cook until the eggs are fully set.

Serve hot for a protein-packed breakfast


Green Smoothie Bowl Ingredients:

1 cup spinach leaves

1/2 ripe avocado

1/2 orange

1/2 cup almond milk

1 tablespoon chia seeds

Fresh berries for topping


Instructions:

Blend spinach, avocado, banana, almond milk, and chia seeds until smooth.

Pour into a bowl and top with fresh berries for extra antioxidants and fiber.

Peanut Butter and Banana Toast Ingredients:

1 slice whole-grain bread

1 tablespoon raw peanut butter

1/2 banana, sliced Cinnamon (optional)

Instructions:

Toast the whole-grain bread.

Spread peanut butter on the toast and top with banana cuts.

Sprinkle with a dash of cinnamon for extra taste

## Lunch and Dinner Creations

Mediterranean Quinoa Salad Ingredients: 1 cup cooked quinoa

1/2 cup chopped cucumber

1/2 cup cherry tomatoes, split

1/4 cup diced red onion

1/4 cup chopped fresh parsley

2 tablespoons olive oil

2 tablespoons lemon juice

Salt and pepper to taste

Crumbled feta cheese (extra)

Instructions:

In a large bowl, mix quinoa, cucumber, cherry tomatoes, red onion, and parsley.

In a small bowl, mix together olive oil and lemon juice. Season with salt and pepper.

Drizzle the dressing over the salad and toss to mix.

If preferred, top with crumbled feta cheese for extra flavor.

Teriyaki Salmon Ingredients:

2 salmon pieces

1/4 cup teriyaki sauce (low-sodium)

2 cloves garlic, minced

1 tablespoon olive oil

Sesame seeds for decoration (optional)

Instructions: In a bowl, mix teriyaki sauce and chopped garlic.

Place salmon pieces in a resealable bag and pour the teriyaki mixture over them. Seal the bag and marinate for 30 minutes.

Heat olive oil in a skillet over medium-high intensity.

Remove fish from the marinade and cook in the skillet for about 4-5 minutes per side, or until the salmon flakes easily.

Garnish with sesame seeds if wanted. Serve with steamed veggies for a balanced meal.

Spaghetti Squash with Pesto and Cherry Tomatoes Ingredients:

1 spaghetti squash, split and seeds removed

2 tablespoons pesto sauce

1 cup cherry tomatoes, sliced

Fresh basil leaves for decoration (optional)

Instructions:

Preheat the oven to 375°F (190°C).

Place the spaghetti squash halves cut-side down on a baking sheet and roast for about 40-45 minutes, or until the squash is tender and easily divided into strands with a fork.

Scrape the squash into strands with a fork and place in a bowl.

Toss the spaghetti squash with pesto sauce and cherry tomatoes.

Garnish with fresh basil leaves for extra taste.

Black Bean Salad Ingredients:

1 can (15 oz) dark beans, depleted and washed

1 cup corn bits (new or frozen, defrosted)

1/2 cup diced red ringer pepper

1/4 cup cleaved new cilantro

Juice of 1 lime

Salt and pepper to taste

Guidelines: In a huge bowl, blend dark beans, corn, diced red ringer pepper, and cilantro.

Sprinkle with lime squeeze and season with salt and pepper.

Toss to mix and serve as a refreshing and fiber-rich salad.

**Snacks and Sides**

Cucumber and Cottage Cheese Slices
Ingredients: 1 cucumber, sliced 1/2 cup low-fat cottage cheese
Fresh dill (optional)
Salt and pepper to taste

Instructions: Arrange cucumber pieces on a plate.

Top each cucumber slice with a spoonful of cottage cheese.

Season with salt, pepper, and fresh dill for added taste.

Mixed Nuts Ingredients:

A handful of mixed nuts (almonds, walnuts, cashews)

Instructions: Enjoy a satisfying and protein-rich snack by getting a handful of mixed nuts. Nuts are a great source of healthy fats and provide long-lasting energy.

Sliced Apple with Almond Butter Ingredients:

1 apple, sliced 2 tbsp almond butter

Instructions: Dip apple slices in almond butter for a satisfying and healthy snack.

# Additional Reading and Tools for Success

1. Books on Intermittent Fasting

A curated list of books that delve deeper into the science and practical parts of intermittent fasting.

2. Fasting Apps and Tools

Recommendations for fasting apps and digital tools to help you in tracking your fasting schedule.

3. Websites and Communities

Links to websites, forums, and online communities where you can find support, help, and inspiration from others on their fasting journeys.